# love letters to my doctors

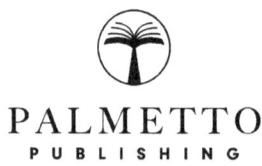

**PALMETTO**
PUBLISHING
Charleston, SC
www.PalmettoPublishing.com

Copyright © 2024
by Rachel Charlton DesRosier

All rights reserved

No portion of this book may be reproduced, stored in a retrieval system, or transmitted in any form by any means–electronic, mechanical, photocopy, recording, etc. - except for brief quotations, with prior permission of the author.

Paperback ISBN: 979-8-8229-4413-8
eBook ISBN: 979-8-8229-4414-5

# love letters to my doctors

**RACHEL CHARLTON DESROSIER**

A true story for your amusement,
your heartbreak, and your healing.

# Preface

I would like this preface to be clear and informative. No long backstory - you will read the whole story at the end of this book. In each of my letters to my doctors, I tell them my diagnosis and the two things that help treat my pain (which I have deleted from the letters in this book since it would be so redundant for you to re-read it in every letter). My chronic pain is caused by faulty brain receptors.

My NMDA receptors are overactive and cause me to perceive pain despite no apparent injury or signs. At this time, the exact details are not known.

The NMDA receptor is a glutamate receptor. Glutamate is the most abundant neurotransmitter in the brain. Basically, my receptors take in too much glutamate. Other substances involved include magnesium and zinc. Perhaps a deficiency of magnesium and/or zinc caused my receptors to be overactive? Maybe the antibiotics (fluoroquinolones) I was given in the hospital caused it? Anyways, the treatment is NMDA antagonists, including dextromethorphan (DXM).

Another pain-killer is the mu-opioid agonist, kratom. Kratom (mitragyna speciosa) is an herb that kept me alive before I found DXM. It is another NMDA antagonist, but not as strong. Kratom has been used by chronic pain sufferers, chronic fatigue sufferers, those with PTSD, and as a treatment for opioid addiction.

Also, Mayonnaise Medical Center diagnosed me with mild POTS (postural orthostatic tachycardia syndrome). For many people, it is debilitating. I am lucky, I just have terrible orthostatic headaches. To my fellow chronic pain people, and my fellow zebras, it is time to unite. Speak your truth. Be your own advocate. And if you find relief and have the spoons, please assist others and advocate for them, too. Love you all.

P.S. - The names of the doctors are obviously changed here to keep them anonymous, but I hope you enjoy the names I came up with. There were more letters than what is included in this book, and yes they were really sent in the mail for Valentine's Day 2024, therefore they are love letters to my doctors.

Side note - Last thing, I promise. As you read the letters you will notice I include the type of doctor they were (cardiologist, neurologist, etc). But none of these are pain management doctors. I went to multiple pain management doctors. Not one of them managed my pain. More about this will be in my next book, *Quality of Life and Death*.

LOVE LETTERS TO MY DOCTORS

To: Dr. Janny Menny,
Psychologist

Hey Jan,

I was a patient of yours for a day many years ago. I am a chronic pain patient and was referred to you by another doctor. I was young and polite back then, now I am getting old and my new year's resolution is to speak my mind more often. I now have a diagnosis which perhaps you should know in case a patient comes your way with the same thing.

This is bittersweet news and I hope you will read this, digest it, and have an open heart. My visit with you was awful. You said things to me including "what exactly would be different in your life if you did not have pain? Sounds like it would not be that different" and "Why don't you try listening to music to distract yourself from the pain?" It was belittling, gaslighting, minimizing. I also needed to discuss the abuse I had endured from doctors who did not believe me, which was ironic because you probably did not believe me. And I could tell that you did not want to talk about that either, so I did not bring it up. At the end of the visit, you asked me to schedule the next appointment. I said something kind, like "oh I do not know my schedule yet" but I knew I would never set foot there again. Not long after this, I contemplated suicide.

Words are weapons. Words are healers. You need to be much more careful with yours.

Love,

Rachel

LOVE LETTERS TO MY DOCTORS

To: Dr. Lacey Prim,
Doctor of Osteopathic Medicine

Hey Dr. Prim,

I came to you as a chronic pain patient and you were very kind. I now have a diagnosis which perhaps you should know in case a patient comes your way with the same thing.

Also, I remember having a little breakdown and crying at my last visit. You were nice, and I asked you to refer me to a psychologist. But the one you referred me to was awful. Please do not refer anyone to her and please be thoughtful when making referrals from now on.

Love,

Rachel

To: Laney Villainey,
Nurse Practitioner

Hey Laney,

I was a patient of yours for a little while. I am a chronic pain patient and asked you to help me. You wanted me to see the local neurologist and I wanted to see another specialist. I needed you to be my ADVOCATE. But you were so blinded by frustration that you became malevolent. The neurologist sat me down and told me he had nothing for me. When I told you this, you called me a quitter (who quit WHOM?) and then I cried and told you that I was frustrated because you were not helping me, and asked you to please help me, please believe me. Then I received a "breakup letter" from your office telling me I was no longer welcome and to find a new doctor.

Here is what the cause of my pain was, in case another patient comes around with the same thing, and perhaps you can actually help a patient for once.

Do better you little bitch! Take that frustration and make it a catalyst for lifting your patients up and advocating for them!

Love,

Rachel

RACHEL CHARLTON DESROSIER

To: Dr. Jimmy John,
Sports Medicine Physician

Hey Jim,

I came to you as a chronic pain patient and you were very kind. I now have a diagnosis which perhaps you should know in case a patient comes your way with the same thing.

I do think more needs to be done in a treatment plan like mine. I remember asking you if I could get a wheelchair. You said no, because I would lose muscle. You had nothing for me. And I know I am not bleeding to death in front of you, but when will quality of life become a priority? I knew you were scared of lawsuits and opioid addictions. But when will potential suicide become a good reason to finally give your chronic pain patient relief from pain?

Love,

Rachel

LOVE LETTERS TO MY DOCTORS

To: Dr. Godfrey Gullible,
Neurologist

Hey God Complex Godfrey,

I came to you as a chronic pain patient and you were rude. I now have a diagnosis which perhaps you should know in case a patient comes your way with the same thing.

Back to you being rude - you talked over me, you acted like I was wasting your time, I tried to give you details in case something was a clue as to what was wrong with me and you said I should only answer the questions you ask. You were a jerk. Do better from now on.

Fuck you,

Rachel

To: Dr. John Nothing,
Cardiologist

Hey Dr. Nothing,

I came to you for a second opinion. Was my pain to be treated by a cardiologist? What the hell was my diagnosis? But you did not have an opinion. I received NO second opinion. You just went "Eh, I trust the cardiologist you already saw." You wasted my time.

Thanks for the nothing you gifted me,

Rachel

## LOVE LETTERS TO MY DOCTORS

To: Dr. Ivan Knowledge

Dear Dr. Knowledge,

This is a long one. Thank you for figuring out my chronic pain. Thank you for believing me, listening, problem-solving, remembering me when I came back for my next visit, thank you for everything. Please feel free to share this with your staff as well - I am hoping some parts might be funny or amusing. At the very least, I hope they feel appreciated - Every phone call they answer, a patient is hopefully closer to getting a diagnosis, getting some relief. I am thankful for them too. Please, whenever you have a hard day, find some humor in it and please also think of my story.

**Backstory**: I was a chubby kid. But by 2009, I was an avid weightlifter and calorie counter. I counted the calories in lettuce! Maybe I had anorexia athletica or something, but nobody would have diagnosed me back then - the adults in my life were just happy I wasn't another chubby teen, so they did not ask questions. I was really starving myself, my reward for working out was a handful of food, and there were a lot of foods that I considered to be "bad" and I remember going on a kayak trip with my family and flipping out because the kayak rental place didn't have bottled water (all the beverages had sugar in them). I probably really needed that sugar! Please give some love to your chubby patients, being fat is not the worst thing a person can be. I was still seeing gains in the weightroom, so I continued my low-calorie diet. I weighed 98 lbs and bench pressed 125 lbs and leg pressed 300 lbs. I got used to feeling hungry. In March 2009, I "craved" heat more than food, I would sit in a car on a hot day to feel better because 90F felt cold. I had a fever. I couldn't keep any food down. I was diagnosed with mononucleosis. My leg muscles would involuntarily twitch/jump and my doctor said it was dehydration. For two weeks, I survived on broth and a few soft foods. At that point, I became so weak I could not walk, could not lift my arms to feed myself so my parents took me to the hospital. My whole body hurt, I was given morphine and had an allergic reaction. I was diagnosed with pneumonia in both lungs, pancreatitis (elevated enzymes, later diagnosed as chronic) and gallbladder disease (no gallstones, just inflamed with 6% ejection fraction, later taken out).

When I was released from the hospital, I was eager to get back into exercise. I forced myself to run. But my body tried to stop me. I had a burning pain from my hips downward whenever I used my legs. Resting gave me some relief. Maybe my body was trying to keep me from exercising too much. For a year, I continued to weight lift and run despite the pain. Then I stopped, I could not take the pain anymore, I was not able to eat or sleep because of the pain and exercising made the pain worse. I joined online anorexia and body dysmorphia support groups, gained weight and stopped calorie counting. Doctors said that maybe the pain was a weird nutritional deficiency symptom, my iron was low and I'd take supplements and eventually my bloodwork got better but the pain remained. I saw neurologists, rheumatologists, sports medicine doctors, pain medicine doctors, gastroenterologists, gynecologists, cardiologists, physical therapists, acupuncturists, etc. Some doctors were good, they believed me and felt for me. Some doctors were awful. They insinuated that I was attention seeking, or drug seeking, or a hypochondriac, or had munchausen syndrome. I had CT scans, PET scans, EKG, EMG, autoimmune marker lab work, veins ablated in my legs, ovarian cyst removed, etc.

Three years into my chronic pain, I was on the verge of losing my college scholarship. I was struggling to walk to classes and was always tardy. My doctor helped me keep my scholarship. Still no answers - we decided it was time to go to the top-ranked hospital in the nation. They were awful. Still no answers. At this point, I knew I would have the pain for the rest of my life. I was surviving - I would have regular breakdowns, but I did not give up. I still went to school, still worked. I tried to will the pain away, think it away, meditate, believe it away. I went to a psychologist - She said "well if you have a job and school and everything, how would your life be different if you didn't have the pain anyway? Have you tried listening to music to distract yourself from the pain?" I started to wonder if death would be a good thing. All this suffering, but not just my own - my parents were so worried about me and they had POURED money into figuring out what was wrong with me. We tried all the wives' tales, all the quack medicine, all the yoga poses, all the specialists, and lots of medications, SSRIs and anticonvulsants with horrible side effects. No doctor ever wanted to give me a prescription pain reliever, but ibuprofen did not touch the pain so maybe it would not have helped anyway. I felt like a burden to the people I loved and wondered what the best way would be to un-alive myself. Death was not scary anymore, it was pain relief.

2012 was a crazy year. Pneumonia again (and later walking pneumonia). I did a few things I shouldn't have, I hated myself. I gave myself an ultimatum - I was either going to find something for my pain so my loved ones did not have to suffer with me so much, or I was going to give myself "the pain relief." This was when I started going to group therapy and invisible illness groups, chronic pain groups, and being around "zebra patients". I listened for supplements, new treatments, medical studies. I was reading medical journals, I was pre-med in college, and applied to PA school but they didn't like my take on how Anthropology is important in the health field (they did not like soft sciences and my degree was Anthropology). Basically, if crack cocaine relieved my pain, I was going to become a crack addict. I found Kratom. Controversial, but it took the edge off. In late 2012, I started dating a wonderful man who would become my husband. He once tasted kratom and threw up. It is like eating mud. But Kratom saved my life! From 2012-2023, it was how I kept alive.

Today is like a miracle. I did not think I would live to see the day where I would get more relief than what Kratom gives me. I know I told you that rest relieves my pain, but now that I have real pain relief I can confirm that I was actually in pain constantly, just different levels of pain. Previous doctors made me feel like I should down-play my pain so I don't seem like a hypochondriac. As of March 2024, I will have had my chronic pain for

15 years. It feels so nice to feel more normal. On my low-pain days, it's almost like I'm a normal person! I'm still feeling kind of shocked, like I must be dreaming/hallucinating. I know I'm not cured, but this is still huge. Thank you for figuring this out for me. Thank you for giving me a new life. I should count the ways:

**Waking up** - Normally, even if I've slept well, I feel pain as soon as my feet hit the ground. Not anymore!

**Breathing** - You know how your body wants to curl up into the fetal position when you're in pain? Try resisting that feeling for 15 years. I once went to a massage therapist who boasted she helped chronic pain sufferers and she kept yelling at me to take deeper breaths - "Slow your breathing and breathe deeper!". I couldn't, I was in so much pain. I am feeling much better now! It feels easier to breathe.

**Cold feet** - Literally. For 15 years, my thighs/legs/feet have felt like they were on fire. I forgot what it feels like to have cold feet. I wear socks and slippers at home now.

**Walking** - I can take a walk in my neighborhood and not feel like there's a nagging burning feeling in half of my body the whole time. You know that feeling when you take your shoes off at the end of a long day and you think "wow it feels so good to take these off"? Multiply it by 100 and that's me taking a short walk.

**Sex** - No details spared, you guys, no details spared. For years, I had sex with my husband and was in pain. Much better now!

**Pooping** - What did I say about no details spared? Sorry not sorry. Kratom gave me constipation. Saving money by not buying kratom and magnesium supplements. Pooping much better now :)

**Loved ones** - My dad cried when I told him about my diagnosis and treatment plan. My mom died of cancer years ago (they think it started in her gallbladder and spread through her digestive system, maybe we have crappy gallbladders in my family). I wish my mom could see this. She always knew how bad my pain was no matter how good of an actor I was. On my wedding day, five minutes into it, I was in pain standing. Nobody knew, but she did. She brought me champagne and encouraged me to sit down. She was a scientist, worked in a laboratory and when she had kids she became a science teacher. But she would still use the word "magic" and used it whenever something amusing or pretty happened, no matter the logical explanation. A rainbow has a reason for its existence, but we enjoy it, therefore it is still "magical" or a "miracle"! I could be dead right now, but a miracle happened. I thought I would be in pain for the rest of my life, but a miracle happened. Thank you.

Again, please feel free to share my story. I hope you are having a good day, and if not, hopefully this letter adds meaningfulness to the day. Thank you for all that you do. Patients can be annoying. Patients be crazy. Please forgive us. Lol.

Sincerely,

Rachel
With the NMDA receptors that don't do right.

www.ingramcontent.com/pod-product-compliance
Lightning Source LLC
LaVergne TN
LVHW051926060526
838201LV00062B/4716